Rock Climbing Log Book

INFORMATIONS

NAME

ADDRESS

E-MAIL ADDRESS

WEBSITE

PHONE   **FAX**

EMERGENCY CONTACT PERSON

PHONE   **FAX**

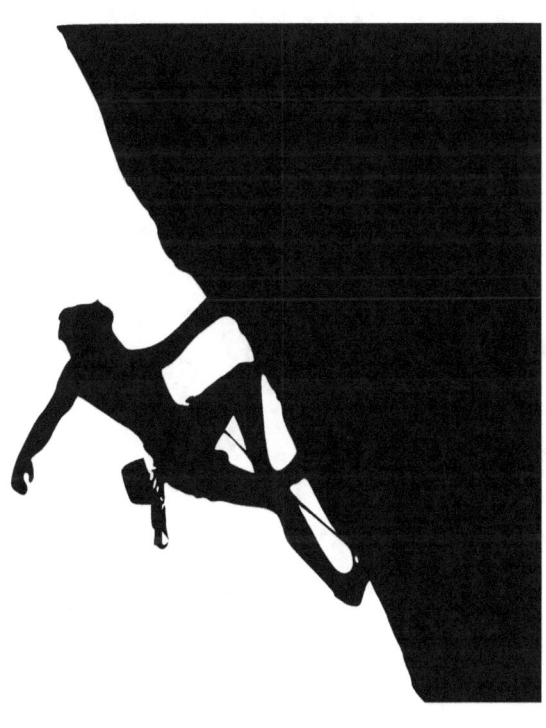

Dedication

This Rock Climbing Journal is dedicated to all the people out there who love rock climbing and want to document their findings in the process.

You are my inspiration for producing books and I'm honored to be a part of keeping all of your rock climbing notes and records organized.

This journal notebook will help you record the details about your rock climbing adventures.

Thoughtfully put together with these sections to record: Name of Climb, Grade, Achieved?, Beta, Attempts, Partners, Strength, Weakness, & Notes.

How to Use this Book

The purpose of this book is to keep all of your Rock Climbing notes all in one place. It will help keep you organized.

This Rock Climbing Journal will allow you to accurately document every detail about your tattoo sketches. It's a great way to chart your course through all of your climbs.

Here are examples of the prompts for you to fill in and write about your experience in this book:

1. Name of Climb - For writing the name of the climb. Also the Date, Style, Location, Routes, and Length.
2. Grade - Record the grade.
3. Achieved? - Write whether you finished the climb.
4. Beta - Log the difficulty, crux, style, length, etc.
5. Attempts - How many attempts did it take you to achieve.
6. Partners - Who did you rock climb with.
7. Strength - What was the one thing you were very good at.
8. Weakness - What was the one thing you need to improve on.
9. Notes - Blank lined space for any additional information such as quality of rock, ease to protect, required equipment, hand or foot holds, best practices detail, ideas for next time, etc.

Rock Climbing Log Book

NAME OF CLIMB

GRADE

DATE

STYLE

ACHIEVED?

LOCATION

ROUTE

LENGTH

BETA

....
....
....
....

ATTEMPTS

PARTNERS

STRENGTH

WEAKNESS

NOTES

....
....
....
....
....

Rock Climbing Log Book

NAME OF CLIMB

GRADE

DATE

STYLE

LOCATION

ACHIEVED?

ROUTE

LENGTH

BETA

....
....
....
....

ATTEMPTS

PARTNERS

STRENGTH

WEAKNESS

NOTES

....
....
....
....
....

Rock Climbing Log Book

NAME OF CLIMB

GRADE

DATE   **STYLE**

LOCATION

ACHIEVED?

ROUTE   **LENGTH**

BETA

....
....
....
....

ATTEMPTS

PARTNERS

STRENGTH

WEAKNESS

NOTES

....
....
....
....
....

Rock Climbing Log Book

NAME OF CLIMB

GRADE

DATE **STYLE**

LOCATION

ACHIEVED?

ROUTE **LENGTH**

BETA

....
....
....
....

ATTEMPTS

PARTNERS

STRENGTH

WEAKNESS

NOTES

....
....
....
....
....

Rock Climbing Log Book

NAME OF CLIMB

GRADE

DATE **STYLE**
LOCATION

ACHIEVED?

ROUTE **LENGTH**

BETA

....
....
....
....

ATTEMPTS

PARTNERS

STRENGTH

WEAKNESS

NOTES

....
....
....
....
....

Rock Climbing Log Book

NAME OF CLIMB

GRADE

DATE STYLE

LOCATION

ACHIEVED?

ROUTE LENGTH

BETA

....
....
....
....

ATTEMPTS

PARTNERS

STRENGTH

WEAKNESS

NOTES

....
....
....
....
....

Rock Climbing Log Book

NAME OF CLIMB

GRADE

DATE

STYLE

ACHIEVED?

LOCATION

ROUTE

LENGTH

BETA

....
....
....
....

ATTEMPTS

PARTNERS

STRENGTH

WEAKNESS

NOTES

....
....
....
....
....

Rock Climbing Log Book

NAME OF CLIMB

GRADE

DATE **STYLE**

LOCATION

ACHIEVED?

ROUTE **LENGTH**

BETA

....
....
....
....

ATTEMPTS

PARTNERS

STRENGTH

WEAKNESS

NOTES

....
....
....
....
....

Rock Climbing Log Book

NAME OF CLIMB

GRADE

DATE   **STYLE**

LOCATION

ACHIEVED?

ROUTE   **LENGTH**

BETA

....
....
....
....

ATTEMPTS

PARTNERS

STRENGTH

WEAKNESS

NOTES

....
....
....
....
....

Rock Climbing Log Book

NAME OF CLIMB

GRADE

DATE STYLE

ACHIEVED?

LOCATION

ROUTE LENGTH

BETA

....
....
....
....

ATTEMPTS

PARTNERS

STRENGTH

WEAKNESS

NOTES

....
....
....
....
....

Rock Climbing Log Book

NAME OF CLIMB

GRADE

DATE   **STYLE**

ACHIEVED?

LOCATION

ROUTE   **LENGTH**

BETA

....
....
....
....

ATTEMPTS

PARTNERS

STRENGTH

WEAKNESS

NOTES

....
....
....
....

Rock Climbing Log Book

NAME OF CLIMB

GRADE

DATE

STYLE

LOCATION

ACHIEVED?

ROUTE

LENGTH

BETA

....
....
....
....

ATTEMPTS

PARTNERS

STRENGTH

WEAKNESS

NOTES

....
....
....
....

Rock Climbing Log Book

NAME OF CLIMB

GRADE

DATE STYLE
LOCATION

ACHIEVED?

ROUTE LENGTH

BETA

....
....
....
....

ATTEMPTS

PARTNERS

STRENGTH

WEAKNESS

NOTES

....
....
....
....
....

Rock Climbing Log Book

NAME OF CLIMB

GRADE

DATE

STYLE

LOCATION

ACHIEVED?

ROUTE

LENGTH

BETA

....
....
....
....

ATTEMPTS

PARTNERS

STRENGTH

WEAKNESS

NOTES

....
....
....
....
....

Rock Climbing Log Book

NAME OF CLIMB

GRADE

DATE STYLE
LOCATION

ACHIEVED?

ROUTE LENGTH

BETA

ATTEMPTS

PARTNERS

STRENGTH

WEAKNESS

NOTES

Rock Climbing Log Book

NAME OF CLIMB

GRADE

DATE

STYLE

LOCATION

ACHIEVED?

ROUTE

LENGTH

BETA

....
....
....
....

ATTEMPTS

PARTNERS

STRENGTH

WEAKNESS

NOTES

....
....
....
....
....

Rock Climbing Log Book

NAME OF CLIMB

GRADE

DATE

STYLE

LOCATION

ACHIEVED?

ROUTE

LENGTH

BETA

....
....
....
....

ATTEMPTS

PARTNERS

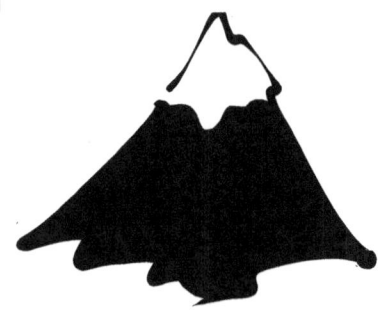

STRENGTH

WEAKNESS

NOTES

....
....
....
....
....

Rock Climbing Log Book

NAME OF CLIMB

GRADE

DATE

STYLE

LOCATION

ACHIEVED?

ROUTE

LENGTH

BETA

....
....
....
....

ATTEMPTS

PARTNERS

STRENGTH

WEAKNESS

NOTES

....
....
....
....
....

Rock Climbing Log Book

NAME OF CLIMB

GRADE

DATE **STYLE**
LOCATION

ACHIEVED?

ROUTE **LENGTH**

BETA

....
....
....
....

ATTEMPTS

PARTNERS

STRENGTH

WEAKNESS

NOTES

....
....
....
....
....

Rock Climbing Log Book

NAME OF CLIMB

GRADE

DATE **STYLE**

LOCATION

ACHIEVED?

ROUTE **LENGTH**

BETA

....
....
....
....

ATTEMPTS

PARTNERS

STRENGTH

WEAKNESS

NOTES

....
....
....
....
....

Rock Climbing Log Book

NAME OF CLIMB	GRADE

DATE　　　　　　STYLE

LOCATION

ACHIEVED?

ROUTE　　　　　　　LENGTH

BETA

....
....
....
....

ATTEMPTS

PARTNERS

STRENGTH	WEAKNESS

NOTES

....
....
....
....
....

Rock Climbing Log Book

NAME OF CLIMB

GRADE

DATE
LOCATION

STYLE

ACHIEVED?

ROUTE
LENGTH

BETA

ATTEMPTS

PARTNERS

STRENGTH

WEAKNESS

NOTES

Rock Climbing Log Book

NAME OF CLIMB

GRADE

DATE

STYLE

LOCATION

ACHIEVED?

ROUTE

LENGTH

BETA

....
....
....
....

ATTEMPTS

PARTNERS

STRENGTH

WEAKNESS

NOTES

....
....
....
....

Rock Climbing Log Book

NAME OF CLIMB

GRADE

DATE STYLE

ACHIEVED?

LOCATION

ROUTE LENGTH

BETA

....
....
....
....

ATTEMPTS

PARTNERS

STRENGTH

WEAKNESS

NOTES

....
....
....
....
....

Rock Climbing Log Book

NAME OF CLIMB

GRADE

DATE

STYLE

ACHIEVED?

LOCATION

ROUTE

LENGTH

BETA

....
....
....
....

ATTEMPTS

PARTNERS

STRENGTH

WEAKNESS

NOTES

....
....
....
....
....

Rock Climbing Log Book

NAME OF CLIMB

GRADE

DATE

STYLE

LOCATION

ACHIEVED?

ROUTE

LENGTH

BETA

....
....
....
....

ATTEMPTS

PARTNERS

STRENGTH

WEAKNESS

NOTES

....
....
....
....
....

Rock Climbing Log Book

NAME OF CLIMB

GRADE

DATE

STYLE

ACHIEVED?

LOCATION

ROUTE

LENGTH

BETA

....
....
....
....

ATTEMPTS

PARTNERS

STRENGTH

WEAKNESS

NOTES

....
....
....
....
....

Rock Climbing Log Book

NAME OF CLIMB

GRADE

DATE

STYLE

LOCATION

ACHIEVED?

ROUTE

LENGTH

BETA

....
....
....
....

ATTEMPTS

PARTNERS

STRENGTH

WEAKNESS

NOTES

....
....
....
....
....

Rock Climbing Log Book

NAME OF CLIMB

GRADE

DATE **STYLE**

LOCATION

ACHIEVED?

ROUTE **LENGTH**

BETA

....
....
....
....

ATTEMPTS

PARTNERS

STRENGTH

WEAKNESS

NOTES

....
....
....
....
....

Rock Climbing Log Book

NAME OF CLIMB

GRADE

DATE STYLE

ACHIEVED?

LOCATION

ROUTE LENGTH

BETA

....
....
....
....

ATTEMPTS

PARTNERS

STRENGTH

WEAKNESS

NOTES

....
....
....
....
....

Rock Climbing Log Book

NAME OF CLIMB

GRADE

DATE STYLE
LOCATION

ACHIEVED?

ROUTE LENGTH

BETA
....
....
....
....

ATTEMPTS

PARTNERS

STRENGTH

WEAKNESS

NOTES
....
....
....
....
....

Rock Climbing Log Book

NAME OF CLIMB

GRADE

DATE

STYLE

ACHIEVED?

LOCATION

ROUTE

LENGTH

BETA

....
....
....
....

ATTEMPTS

PARTNERS

STRENGTH

WEAKNESS

NOTES

....
....
....
....
....
....

Rock Climbing Log Book

NAME OF CLIMB

GRADE

DATE **STYLE**
LOCATION

ACHIEVED?

ROUTE **LENGTH**

BETA

....
....
....
....

ATTEMPTS

PARTNERS

STRENGTH

WEAKNESS

NOTES

....
....
....
....
....

Rock Climbing Log Book

NAME OF CLIMB

GRADE

DATE
LOCATION
STYLE

ACHIEVED?

ROUTE
LENGTH

BETA

....
....
....
....

ATTEMPTS

PARTNERS

STRENGTH

WEAKNESS

NOTES

....
....
....
....
....

Rock Climbing Log Book

NAME OF CLIMB

GRADE

DATE STYLE

LOCATION

ACHIEVED?

ROUTE LENGTH

BETA

....
....
....
....

ATTEMPTS

PARTNERS

STRENGTH

WEAKNESS

NOTES

....
....
....
....
....

Rock Climbing Log Book

NAME OF CLIMB

GRADE

DATE

STYLE

ACHIEVED?

LOCATION

ROUTE

LENGTH

BETA

....
....
....
....

ATTEMPTS

PARTNERS

STRENGTH

WEAKNESS

NOTES

....
....
....
....
....

Rock Climbing Log Book

NAME OF CLIMB

GRADE

DATE

STYLE

LOCATION

ACHIEVED?

ROUTE

LENGTH

BETA

....
....
....
....

ATTEMPTS

PARTNERS

STRENGTH

WEAKNESS

NOTES

....
....
....
....
....

Rock Climbing Log Book

NAME OF CLIMB

GRADE

DATE **STYLE**

LOCATION

ACHIEVED?

ROUTE **LENGTH**

BETA

....
....
....
....

ATTEMPTS

PARTNERS

STRENGTH

WEAKNESS

NOTES

....
....
....
....
....

Rock Climbing Log Book

NAME OF CLIMB

GRADE

DATE STYLE

LOCATION

ACHIEVED?

ROUTE LENGTH

BETA

....
....
....
....

ATTEMPTS

PARTNERS

STRENGTH

WEAKNESS

NOTES

....
....
....
....
....

Rock Climbing Log Book

NAME OF CLIMB

GRADE

DATE

STYLE

ACHIEVED?

LOCATION

ROUTE

LENGTH

BETA

....
....
....
....

ATTEMPTS

PARTNERS

STRENGTH

WEAKNESS

NOTES

....
....
....
....
....

Rock Climbing Log Book

NAME OF CLIMB

GRADE

DATE **STYLE**

LOCATION

ACHIEVED?

ROUTE **LENGTH**

BETA

ATTEMPTS

PARTNERS

STRENGTH

WEAKNESS

NOTES

Rock Climbing Log Book

NAME OF CLIMB

GRADE

DATE **STYLE**

ACHIEVED?

LOCATION

ROUTE **LENGTH**

BETA

....
....
....
....

ATTEMPTS

PARTNERS

STRENGTH

WEAKNESS

NOTES

....
....
....
....
....

Rock Climbing Log Book

NAME OF CLIMB

GRADE

DATE

STYLE

LOCATION

ACHIEVED?

ROUTE

LENGTH

BETA

....
....
....
....

ATTEMPTS

PARTNERS

STRENGTH

WEAKNESS

NOTES

....
....
....
....
....

Rock Climbing Log Book

NAME OF CLIMB

GRADE

DATE

STYLE

LOCATION

ACHIEVED?

ROUTE

LENGTH

BETA

....
....
....
....

ATTEMPTS

PARTNERS

STRENGTH

WEAKNESS

NOTES

....
....
....
....
....

Rock Climbing Log Book

NAME OF CLIMB

GRADE

DATE

STYLE

LOCATION

ACHIEVED?

ROUTE

LENGTH

BETA

ATTEMPTS

PARTNERS

STRENGTH

WEAKNESS

NOTES

Rock Climbing Log Book

NAME OF CLIMB

GRADE

DATE **STYLE**

LOCATION

ACHIEVED?

ROUTE **LENGTH**

BETA

....
....
....
....

ATTEMPTS

PARTNERS

STRENGTH

WEAKNESS

NOTES

....
....
....
....
....

Rock Climbing Log Book

NAME OF CLIMB

GRADE

DATE STYLE
LOCATION

ACHIEVED?

ROUTE LENGTH

BETA

....
....
....
....

ATTEMPTS

PARTNERS

STRENGTH

WEAKNESS

NOTES

....
....
....
....
....

Rock Climbing Log Book

NAME OF CLIMB

GRADE

DATE **STYLE**

LOCATION

ACHIEVED?

ROUTE **LENGTH**

BETA

....
....
....
....

ATTEMPTS

PARTNERS

STRENGTH

WEAKNESS

NOTES

....
....
....
....
....

Rock Climbing Log Book

NAME OF CLIMB	GRADE

DATE   STYLE

LOCATION

ACHIEVED?

ROUTE   LENGTH

BETA

....
....
....
....

ATTEMPTS

PARTNERS

STRENGTH

WEAKNESS

NOTES

....
....
....
....

Rock Climbing Log Book

NAME OF CLIMB

GRADE

DATE **STYLE**

LOCATION

ACHIEVED?

ROUTE **LENGTH**

BETA

....
....
....
....

ATTEMPTS

PARTNERS

STRENGTH

WEAKNESS

NOTES

....
....
....
....

Rock Climbing Log Book

NAME OF CLIMB

GRADE

DATE **STYLE**

LOCATION

ACHIEVED?

ROUTE **LENGTH**

BETA

ATTEMPTS

PARTNERS

STRENGTH

WEAKNESS

NOTES

Rock Climbing Log Book

NAME OF CLIMB

GRADE

DATE

STYLE

LOCATION

ACHIEVED?

ROUTE

LENGTH

BETA

....
....
....
....

ATTEMPTS

PARTNERS

STRENGTH

WEAKNESS

NOTES

....
....
....
....
....

Rock Climbing Log Book

NAME OF CLIMB

GRADE

DATE　　　　　　　STYLE

LOCATION

ACHIEVED?

ROUTE　　　　　　　LENGTH

BETA

....
....
....
....

ATTEMPTS

PARTNERS

STRENGTH

WEAKNESS

NOTES

....
....
....
....
....

Rock Climbing Log Book

NAME OF CLIMB

GRADE

DATE STYLE

LOCATION

ACHIEVED?

ROUTE LENGTH

BETA

....
....
....
....

ATTEMPTS

PARTNERS

STRENGTH

WEAKNESS

NOTES

....
....
....
....
....

Rock Climbing Log Book

NAME OF CLIMB

GRADE

DATE

STYLE

LOCATION

ACHIEVED?

ROUTE

LENGTH

BETA

....
....
....
....

ATTEMPTS

PARTNERS

STRENGTH

WEAKNESS

NOTES

....
....
....
....
....

Rock Climbing Log Book

NAME OF CLIMB

GRADE

DATE

STYLE

ACHIEVED?

LOCATION

ROUTE

LENGTH

BETA

....
....
....
....

ATTEMPTS

PARTNERS

STRENGTH

WEAKNESS

NOTES

....
....
....
....
....

Rock Climbing Log Book

NAME OF CLIMB

GRADE

DATE STYLE
LOCATION

ACHIEVED?

ROUTE LENGTH

BETA

ATTEMPTS

PARTNERS

STRENGTH

WEAKNESS

NOTES

Rock Climbing Log Book

NAME OF CLIMB

GRADE

DATE **STYLE**

LOCATION

ACHIEVED?

ROUTE **LENGTH**

BETA

....
....
....
....

ATTEMPTS

PARTNERS

STRENGTH

WEAKNESS

NOTES

....
....
....
....
....

Rock Climbing Log Book

NAME OF CLIMB

GRADE

DATE   STYLE

LOCATION

ACHIEVED?

ROUTE   LENGTH

BETA

....
....
....

ATTEMPTS

PARTNERS

STRENGTH

WEAKNESS

NOTES

....
....
....
....
....

Rock Climbing Log Book

NAME OF CLIMB

GRADE

DATE

STYLE

ACHIEVED?

LOCATION

ROUTE

LENGTH

BETA

....
....
....
....

ATTEMPTS

PARTNERS

STRENGTH

WEAKNESS

NOTES

....
....
....
....
....

Rock Climbing Log Book

NAME OF CLIMB

GRADE

DATE　　　　　　　STYLE

LOCATION

ACHIEVED?

ROUTE　　　　　　　LENGTH

BETA

....
....
....
....

ATTEMPTS

PARTNERS

STRENGTH

WEAKNESS

NOTES

....
....
....
....
....

Rock Climbing Log Book

NAME OF CLIMB

GRADE

DATE

STYLE

LOCATION

ACHIEVED?

ROUTE

LENGTH

BETA

....
....
....
....

ATTEMPTS

PARTNERS

STRENGTH

WEAKNESS

NOTES

....
....
....
....
....

Rock Climbing Log Book

NAME OF CLIMB

GRADE

DATE   STYLE

LOCATION

ACHIEVED?

ROUTE   LENGTH

BETA

....
....
....
....

ATTEMPTS

PARTNERS

STRENGTH

WEAKNESS

NOTES

....
....
....
....
....
....

Rock Climbing Log Book

NAME OF CLIMB

GRADE

DATE

STYLE

ACHIEVED?

LOCATION

ROUTE

LENGTH

BETA

....
....
....
....

ATTEMPTS

PARTNERS

STRENGTH

WEAKNESS

NOTES

....
....
....
....
....

Rock Climbing Log Book

NAME OF CLIMB	GRADE

DATE STYLE

LOCATION

ACHIEVED?

ROUTE LENGTH

BETA
....
....
....
....

ATTEMPTS

PARTNERS

STRENGTH	WEAKNESS

NOTES
....
....
....
....
....

Rock Climbing Log Book

NAME OF CLIMB

GRADE

DATE **STYLE**

LOCATION

ACHIEVED?

ROUTE **LENGTH**

BETA

....
....
....
....

ATTEMPTS

PARTNERS

STRENGTH

WEAKNESS

NOTES

....
....
....
....
....

Rock Climbing Log Book

NAME OF CLIMB

GRADE

DATE STYLE
LOCATION

ACHIEVED?

ROUTE LENGTH

BETA

....
....
....
....

ATTEMPTS

PARTNERS

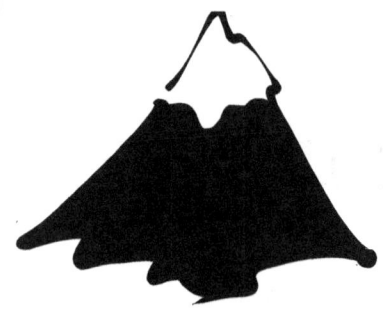

STRENGTH

WEAKNESS

NOTES

....
....
....
....
....

Rock Climbing Log Book

NAME OF CLIMB

GRADE

DATE　　　　　**STYLE**

LOCATION

ACHIEVED?

ROUTE　　　　　**LENGTH**

BETA

....
....
....
....

ATTEMPTS

PARTNERS

STRENGTH

WEAKNESS

NOTES

....
....
....
....
....

Rock Climbing Log Book

NAME OF CLIMB	GRADE

DATE STYLE
LOCATION

ACHIEVED?

ROUTE LENGTH

BETA

....
....
....
....

ATTEMPTS

PARTNERS

STRENGTH	WEAKNESS

NOTES

....
....
....
....
....

Rock Climbing Log Book

NAME OF CLIMB

GRADE

DATE

STYLE

ACHIEVED?

LOCATION

ROUTE

LENGTH

BETA

....
....
....
....

ATTEMPTS

PARTNERS

STRENGTH

WEAKNESS

NOTES

....
....
....
....
....

Rock Climbing Log Book

NAME OF CLIMB

GRADE

DATE STYLE
LOCATION

ACHIEVED?

ROUTE LENGTH

BETA

....
....
....
....

ATTEMPTS

PARTNERS

STRENGTH

WEAKNESS

NOTES

....
....
....
....
....

Rock Climbing Log Book

NAME OF CLIMB

GRADE

DATE

STYLE

ACHIEVED?

LOCATION

ROUTE

LENGTH

BETA

....
....
....
....

ATTEMPTS

PARTNERS

STRENGTH

WEAKNESS

NOTES

....
....
....
....
....

Rock Climbing Log Book

NAME OF CLIMB

GRADE

DATE   STYLE

LOCATION

ACHIEVED?

ROUTE   LENGTH

BETA

....
....
....
....

ATTEMPTS

PARTNERS

STRENGTH

WEAKNESS

NOTES

....
....
....
....
....

Rock Climbing Log Book

NAME OF CLIMB

GRADE

DATE

STYLE

LOCATION

ACHIEVED?

ROUTE

LENGTH

BETA

....
....
....
....

ATTEMPTS

PARTNERS

STRENGTH

WEAKNESS

NOTES

....
....
....
....
....
....

Rock Climbing Log Book

NAME OF CLIMB

GRADE

DATE   STYLE

LOCATION

ACHIEVED?

ROUTE   LENGTH

BETA

ATTEMPTS

PARTNERS

STRENGTH

WEAKNESS

NOTES

Rock Climbing Log Book

NAME OF CLIMB

GRADE

DATE **STYLE**

LOCATION

ACHIEVED?

ROUTE **LENGTH**

BETA

....
....
....
....

ATTEMPTS

PARTNERS

STRENGTH

WEAKNESS

NOTES

....
....
....
....
....

Rock Climbing Log Book

NAME OF CLIMB

GRADE

DATE STYLE
LOCATION

ACHIEVED?

ROUTE LENGTH

BETA

....
....
....
....

ATTEMPTS

PARTNERS

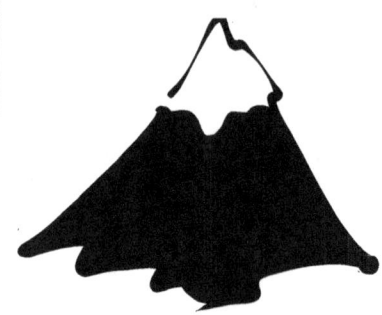

STRENGTH

WEAKNESS

NOTES

....
....
....
....

Rock Climbing Log Book

NAME OF CLIMB

GRADE

DATE   **STYLE**

LOCATION

ACHIEVED?

ROUTE   **LENGTH**

BETA

....
....
....
....

ATTEMPTS

PARTNERS

STRENGTH

WEAKNESS

NOTES

....
....
....
....
....

Rock Climbing Log Book

NAME OF CLIMB

GRADE

DATE　　　　　　　STYLE

LOCATION

ACHIEVED?

ROUTE　　　　　　　LENGTH

BETA

....
....
....
....

ATTEMPTS

PARTNERS

STRENGTH

WEAKNESS

NOTES

....
....
....
....
....

Rock Climbing Log Book

NAME OF CLIMB

GRADE

DATE **STYLE**

LOCATION

ACHIEVED?

ROUTE **LENGTH**

BETA

....
....
....
....

ATTEMPTS

PARTNERS

STRENGTH

WEAKNESS

NOTES

....
....
....
....
....

Rock Climbing Log Book

NAME OF CLIMB

GRADE

DATE STYLE
LOCATION

ACHIEVED?

ROUTE LENGTH

BETA

....
....
....
....

ATTEMPTS

PARTNERS

STRENGTH

WEAKNESS

NOTES

....
....
....
....
....

Rock Climbing Log Book

NAME OF CLIMB

GRADE

DATE　　　　　**STYLE**

ACHIEVED?

LOCATION

ROUTE　　　　　**LENGTH**

BETA

....
....
....
....

ATTEMPTS

PARTNERS

STRENGTH

WEAKNESS

NOTES

....
....
....
....
....

Rock Climbing Log Book

NAME OF CLIMB

GRADE

DATE STYLE

LOCATION

ACHIEVED?

ROUTE LENGTH

BETA

....
....
....
....

ATTEMPTS

PARTNERS

STRENGTH

WEAKNESS

NOTES

....
....
....
....
....

Rock Climbing Log Book

NAME OF CLIMB

GRADE

DATE

STYLE

LOCATION

ACHIEVED?

ROUTE

LENGTH

BETA

....
....
....
....

ATTEMPTS

PARTNERS

STRENGTH

WEAKNESS

NOTES

....
....
....
....
....

Rock Climbing Log Book

NAME OF CLIMB

GRADE

DATE **STYLE**

LOCATION

ACHIEVED?

ROUTE **LENGTH**

BETA

ATTEMPTS

PARTNERS

STRENGTH

WEAKNESS

NOTES

Rock Climbing Log Book

NAME OF CLIMB

GRADE

DATE

STYLE

LOCATION

ACHIEVED?

ROUTE

LENGTH

BETA

....
....
....
....

ATTEMPTS

PARTNERS

STRENGTH

WEAKNESS

NOTES

....
....
....
....
....

Rock Climbing Log Book

NAME OF CLIMB	GRADE

DATE STYLE

LOCATION

	ACHIEVED?

ROUTE LENGTH

BETA

....
....
....
....

ATTEMPTS

PARTNERS

STRENGTH	WEAKNESS

NOTES

....
....
....
....
....

Rock Climbing Log Book

NAME OF CLIMB

GRADE

DATE   **STYLE**

ACHIEVED?

LOCATION

ROUTE   **LENGTH**

BETA
....
....
....
....

ATTEMPTS

PARTNERS

STRENGTH

WEAKNESS

NOTES
....
....
....
....
....

Rock Climbing Log Book

NAME OF CLIMB

GRADE

DATE **STYLE**

LOCATION

ACHIEVED?

ROUTE **LENGTH**

BETA

....
....
....
....

ATTEMPTS

PARTNERS

STRENGTH

WEAKNESS

NOTES

....
....
....
....
....

Rock Climbing Log Book

NAME OF CLIMB

GRADE

DATE

STYLE

LOCATION

ACHIEVED?

ROUTE

LENGTH

BETA

....
....
....
....

ATTEMPTS

PARTNERS

STRENGTH

WEAKNESS

NOTES

....
....
....
....
....

Rock Climbing Log Book

NAME OF CLIMB

GRADE

DATE   STYLE

LOCATION

ACHIEVED?

ROUTE   LENGTH

BETA

....
....
....
....

ATTEMPTS

PARTNERS

STRENGTH

WEAKNESS

NOTES

....
....
....
....
....

Rock Climbing Log Book

NAME OF CLIMB

GRADE

DATE

STYLE

LOCATION

ACHIEVED?

ROUTE

LENGTH

BETA

....
....
....
....

ATTEMPTS

PARTNERS

STRENGTH

WEAKNESS

NOTES

....
....
....
....
....

Rock Climbing Log Book

NAME OF CLIMB

GRADE

DATE **STYLE**

LOCATION

ACHIEVED?

ROUTE **LENGTH**

BETA

ATTEMPTS

PARTNERS

STRENGTH

WEAKNESS

NOTES

Rock Climbing Log Book

NAME OF CLIMB

GRADE

DATE STYLE

LOCATION

ACHIEVED?

ROUTE LENGTH

BETA

....
....
....
....

ATTEMPTS

PARTNERS

STRENGTH

WEAKNESS

NOTES

....
....
....
....
....

Rock Climbing Log Book

NAME OF CLIMB

GRADE

DATE   STYLE

LOCATION

ACHIEVED?

ROUTE   LENGTH

BETA

....
....
....
....

ATTEMPTS

PARTNERS

STRENGTH

WEAKNESS

NOTES

....
....
....
....
....

Rock Climbing Log Book

NAME OF CLIMB

GRADE

DATE

STYLE

ACHIEVED?

LOCATION

ROUTE

LENGTH

BETA

....
....
....
....

ATTEMPTS

PARTNERS

STRENGTH

WEAKNESS

NOTES

....
....
....
....
....

Rock Climbing Log Book

NAME OF CLIMB

GRADE

DATE   STYLE

LOCATION

ACHIEVED?

ROUTE   LENGTH

BETA

....
....
....
....

ATTEMPTS

PARTNERS

STRENGTH

WEAKNESS

NOTES

....
....
....
....
....

Rock Climbing Log Book

NAME OF CLIMB

GRADE

DATE

STYLE

LOCATION

ACHIEVED?

ROUTE

LENGTH

BETA

....
....
....
....

ATTEMPTS

PARTNERS

STRENGTH

WEAKNESS

NOTES

....
....
....
....
....

Rock Climbing Log Book

NAME OF CLIMB

GRADE

DATE　　　　　　STYLE

LOCATION

ACHIEVED?

ROUTE　　　　　　LENGTH

BETA

ATTEMPTS

PARTNERS

STRENGTH

WEAKNESS

NOTES

www.ingramcontent.com/pod-product-compliance
Lightning Source LLC
Chambersburg PA
CBHW071406080526
44587CB00017B/3187